HEALING WITH
Bach Flower Mandalas

ALSO BY GUDRUN PENSELIN

*Healing Spirituality—A Practical Guide to Understanding
and Working with Bach Flowers*
A comprehensive, practical guide and working tool for the implementation of Bach Flower's into a person's daily life.

Bach Flowers Unfolding
A set of cards and a booklet with instructions on how to use Bach
Flower Remedies.

*Herbal Pharmacy for Everyone—A Step-by-Step Guide
to Creating Your Own Herbal Preparations*
Instructional DVD with subtitles in English, French, Spanish and German

HEALING WITH
Bach Flower Mandalas

GUDRUN PENSELIN, M.ED.

Clinical Herbal Therapist, Bach Flower Practitioner

Illustrations by YANA-LEE KRATSCHAT

Rainbow Healing Publishing
R.R.#1, Site 1, Box 11
Wembley, AB
Canada

www.rainbowhealing.ca

ISBN 978-0-9684108-3-7

First edition 2016

Designed by AuthorSupport.com

Original art by Yana-Lee Kratschat

Cover art: Kay Marie Enns. Copyright © 1998-2016 Rainbow Healing Publishing

Library and Archives of Canada Cataloguing in Publication is available upon request.

I dedicate this book to Mother Earth, the children of this Earth, who are our future, and in particular, to my granddaughter Vera, who brings hope and light with her joyful spirit for the healing of this planet and humankind.

"The flowers of tomorrow are in the seeds of today."

~AUTHOR UNKNOWN

Contents

Acknowledgements

I thank my friends who inspired and encouraged me with their enthusiasm to make *Healing with Bach Flower Mandalas* a reality. A very special thank you to my daughter Yana-Lee. Without her this book would not have been possible. While raising her young family Yana-Lee shared her artistic talent in the creation of the illustrations which adds a special touch to the book through her wonderful spirit. Thank you to Catherine for her support with her insightful editing skills. Thank you to all of you who have, knowingly or unknowingly, supported me on my journey and given me the courage and encouragement to step out further into the public light.

Preface

The seed for the creation of *Healing with Bach Flower Mandalas* was planted by my daughter Lena and numerous friends who "nudged me gently" to develop this work which follows the recently published book *Healing Spirituality - A Practical Guide to Understanding and Working with Bach Flowers*.

Healing with Bach Flower Mandalas can be considered a fun tool for working with Bach Flowers. This book is much more than just another mandala colouring book. The combination of Bach Flowers and mandalas provides vast potential and opportunity for healing, movement and transformation. The intent put forth during the creation of this text and art makes *Healing with Bach Flower Mandalas* even more powerful. Designing and colouring the Bach Flower mandalas can be enjoyed by anyone regardless of a person's "artistic" skill level; there is no right or wrong, every creation is perfect the way it is. The book can be used on its own or as a valuable adjunct to any form of Bach Flower therapy including working with the cards from *Bach Flowers Unfolding*. (See the appendix for more information about *Bach Flowers Unfolding*.)

Introduction

"We have been created to love and to be loved."

~ MOTHER TERESA

Healing with Bach Flower Mandalas provides a unique opportunity to explore the potential for transformation and healing through the combination of colour, design and nature in the form of mandalas and Bach Flowers.

Explore the power of colouring Bach Flower mandalas and become part of your own healing journey. These mandalas assist you in freeing yourself of limitations which may hold you back from becoming all who you are meant to be. Working with Bach Flower mandalas may transform fears into courage. The activity may encourage you to focus your life on the present instead of dreaming of a better future or hanging on to the past. Feelings of inadequacies may dissolve. Watch your life unfold in a fun and playful way as you discover the beautiful and dynamic dance between Bach Flowers, colour, form and mandalas as they are intricately and harmoniously interwoven with each other. All are subtle and gentle yet powerful tools of vibrational healing that can have a profound effect on all levels of our being–emotional, spiritual, mental and physical.

It is necessary to actually experience the power of working with mandalas in order to be able to fully grasp their immense potential for healing and transformation.

With this book you hold in your hands the "flowers" that developed from the seeds that were planted by some of my friends but also long before by Edward Bach through the creation of the system of healing known today as the Bach Flower remedies. I hope that, regardless of your intent (fun or conscious therapy), you will enjoy the experience as you tap into your inner self and allow your creativity to flow, leading to inner peace, balance and harmony. May you receive guidance, clarity and inspiration from immersing yourself in the wonderful and mystical world of Bach Flower mandalas. Watch restrictions and limitations melt away gently, encouraging you to live your life with joy in accordance with your Soul.

Chapter 1

Edward Bach and Bach Flowers

"The action of these remedies is to raise our vibrations and open up our channels for the reception of our Spiritual Self, to flood our natures with the particular virtue we need, and wash out from us the fault which is causing harm."

~EDWARD BACH

Edward Bach was born in Moseley, near Birmingham, England on September 24, 1886 and passed on November 27, 1936 at the age of 50. During his childhood he expressed an exceptional love and deep connection to all of nature accompanied by the strong desire to ease suffering. This lead him to eventually study medicine and become a doctor and bacteriologist while at the same time realizing that practical experience and astute observation of patients and people were much more important than studying from books. He considered his intuition and practical experience to be his most valuable teachers in life.

Even though Edward Bach was extremely successful in his practice and research he felt dissatisfied with many aspects of conventional medicine. He recognized many of its limitations and disagreed with the symptomatic approach of primarily relieving and suppressing symptoms rather than providing true healing. He was driven to find a form of medicine that was more gentle, painless, benign and effective in providing long-lasting healing. In his search for such a form of medicine he soon realized that the success of a treatment was strongly influenced by the personality of the individual. This meant that treating the

1

person as a whole was a prerequisite for the possibility of true healing rather than focusing on the dis-ease and its symptoms alone. Even though Bach was aware of the importance of taking care of our bodies in the purely physical form by providing proper nutrition, rest, fresh air and exposure to sun light, according to him physical ailments were primarily the result of imbalances in the emotional, spiritual and mental aspects of our being.

"Health depends on being in harmony with our souls."

~Edward Bach

Guided by his strong intuition and connection to spirit he returned to nature to discover the healing powers of the plants which ultimately lead to the development of what is known today as the Bach Flower remedies. Bach Flower essences can be classified as a form of vibrational healing which are very gentle yet effective and powerful at the same time. They are made from specific blooms of flowering plants and trees. The Bach Flower system is comprised of 38 individual flower essences plus the Rescue Remedy, a combination of five of the individual flower essences.

For more stories of the life of Edward Bach, his philosophy about life and healing and the Bach Flowers, please refer to the book *Healing Spirituality–A Practical Guide to Understanding and Working with Bach Flowers* by Gudrun Penselin. (See appendix for more information about this book.)

Chapter 2

Mandalas General Information

"Healing and freedom from suffering–on a personal and global scale–is in direct proportion to our ability to return to the harmony and understanding of this sacred circle of life. This since the very beginning, has been the practice of creating mandalas."

~Judith Cornell

Mandalas have been part of Hindu and Buddhist cultures for thousands of years. They have been used in the performance of sacred rites and as a medium for meditation. The word *mandala* originates from Sanskrit and means *circle*. The circle is the most common universal sign and found in all cultures around the world. It has no beginning or end and represents the universe, wholeness, the infinite, eternity, and the self and Soul. Mandalas reflect the cycles of the seasons and nature. In native American traditions the Medicine Wheel is used as a mandala. It is seen as the sacred circle or sacred hoop of life which contains all of life and is closely connected to nature. Mandala traditions reflect experiences of life and truth. They have been used as a medium to connect to spirit, one's Soul essence and to help understand and discover the essence of life.

Mandalas can take on many different forms: a circular garden, an arrangement of stones or flowers, patterns drawn in sand, sketches on a piece of paper as well as walking a labyrinth. You can even create mandalas by stirring your soup in circular motions. Once you awaken to the wonderful and beautiful world of mandalas you will find them everywhere and realize how much they are part of creation and our every day living.

The mandalas you create are a reflection of your inner world. It is a process that symbolizes your mental, emotional, spiritual and physical self and is a form of communication between the conscious and subconscious. Working with mandalas facilitates possibilities to reconnect to our Higher Self and Soul and allows us to gain self knowledge, find guidance and direction in life. This meditative activity instills a sense of calmness, contentment and peace, encouraging a person to be still and present in the moment. When we live in the present our mind cannot dwell on the past or be concerned about the future, allowing us to let go of troubling thoughts and emotions. Creating and colouring mandalas is relaxing and grounding, helps to ease stress and anxiety and at times can lead to powerful experiences resulting in long-lasting personal transformation and healing.

Chapter 3

EXPLORE

Healing with Bach Flower Mandalas

"In silence we will find new energy and true unity. Silence gives us a new outlook."

~MOTHER TERESA

Creating and colouring mandalas can take on many different forms, it very much is a personal experience. As such there are no rules as to how to go about this practice or when to get involved. There is no need to wait until moments of stress or crisis in order to be able to enjoy the practice and benefits of designing mandalas. The most important thing is that you enjoy the experience and allow yourself to follow your intuition in every aspect such as the choice of mandala, colours and medium (pencil crayons, markers, coloured sand, dried flowers etc.). Be spontaneous, have fun and trust in the process. Regardless of your preferences, each time you work with the Bach Flower mandalas in this book your life will be enriched and be effected in some positive way. Even if you are not conscious of the changes, you can be assured that a healing shift has occurred, allowing you to move forward in your life with more ease.

The essence of each respective Bach Flower is contained within the mandalas and its healing support is brought forth as you immerse yourself in this activity. The ultimate goal of working with Bach Flowers is to assist us in getting closer to our Soul which results in a better understanding of our path and purpose in life. As part of this journey Bach Flowers are a great means of freeing ourselves from limiting emotions and beliefs. Combining this potential with mandalas increases the possibilities for transformation exponentially.

General Guidelines

- Keep your experience "light", have fun playing with colour, medium and form. Explore in a care free way like a child.
- Allow yourself to add your own designs; nobody says you have to stay within the lines.
- Remember, there is no right or wrong, every creation is perfect and beautiful and is a reflection of your personal journey and where you are at in your life in this moment in time.
- Your approach to working with this book will differ depending on your goals and intentions. If you are looking for spiritual guidance or answers to specific questions and circumstances your practice will most likely be different compared to creating a mandala out of pure enjoyment or for the purpose of relaxation.
- Working with mandalas is effective when done as an individual or group activity.
- Colouring mandalas can be done in many different situations, for example while travelling, listening to a lecture or as a relaxing activity before going to bed.
- Some people like to create a quiet, or even sacred space that allows them to move into a meditative state before engaging with the mandala. Others may not engage in any specific preparations. It is a matter of individual choices.
- Lighting a candle, incense and/or playing soft music will help generate a favourable environment and enhance the ability to connect to deeper levels of our consciousness and our Higher Self.
- Creating mandalas is applied as therapeutic practice in areas of social work, mental health, addiction counselling, abuse, crisis and trauma work and schools.
- Remember to trust and do what feels right and comfortable for you.

Specific Suggestions

OPTION 1:

- Pick a design you are most drawn to, allow your artistic spirit to flow and have fun colouring and creating your mandala. You may want to use the *Reflections* page to journal your experiences.

OPTION 2:

- Get organized by creating your space and gathering all the materials you want to use.
- When you are ready close your eyes, take a few deep breaths and calm your mind.

- Acknowledge your thoughts and emotions. Make a mental note of how you are feeling–emotionally, mentally, physically and spiritually. You may want to rate some of your sensations on a scale of 1 to 10 and write them down on the reflections page, another journal or simply a sheet of paper. For example: headache–5, sadness–8 and so on.

- Focus on a question or circumstance you would like to gain insight, clarity, guidance, support and/or healing with. The questions can be very specific and relate to minute situations or they can take on a much broader even more philosophical context such as: What is the meaning of life? The importance lies in clearly formulating your intention.

- When you feel ready choose an image from *Healing with Bach Flower Mandalas*. You can do this by simply opening the book and work with that mandala or you can choose one by browsing through the images and select the one that you feel drawn to.

- Once you have decided on the illustration, you may want to look or gaze at it first and observe if this elicits any emotions, thoughts or physical sensations. You may decide to make a few notes about your reactions.

- Since you are working with a Bach Flower mandala you may also ask the spirit of the specific Bach Flower to come forward and join you in this healing, transformational exercise while at the same time expressing gratitude to the spirit of the flower for her willingness to share and support you.

- Whenever you feel ready, begin playing with colour, form and medium. Immerse yourself and truly go with the flow, allowing your creativity to blossom and express itself freely. Allow any emotions to surface including tears–remember every tear is a healing tear–and embrace the experience with an open mind and heart. Expect the unexpected. Stay with it until you get a sense of completion. Thank the spirit of the flower again for having come into your life.

Reflections

- Journal about your experience, write, draw or maybe create your own mandala on the *Reflections* page. You may also choose to share your experiences with a friend. Sharing either in the form of journaling or with someone is important because it facilitates and amplifies the potential for change and healing.

- Ask yourself: How am I feeling now? Are there any changes compared to before I created the Bach Flower mandala and if yes, how would I rate them now? Did any emotions shift or surface? Do I have more clarity? Does my spirit feel awakened or do I feel a stronger sense of being connected to the Earth? Did I have a revelation or get a message? Am I feeling inspired, empowered, relieved....?

- You may choose to reflect on your colour choices. What colours did you use or not use? What meaning do the colours have to you personally? You may want to research the meaning of different colours.

- Work with the message of the Bach Flower by using it as an affirmation.
- Learn more about the meaning of the Bach Flower that you have chosen and integrate it into your life. (See the appendix for resources).

Most important of all is that you enjoy your time as you enter into "communication" with these Bach Flower mandalas and access deeper levels of consciousness. Creating and colouring Bach Flower mandalas encourages us to get closer to our Soul and guides us in strengthening our connection to the Earth, both required for our own healing and the healing of Mother Earth.

Chapter 4

Bach Flower Mandalas

"The future does not just happen, it is created. Our destiny is not in the stars, but within ourselves."

~AUTHOR UNKNOWN

Each mandala in this book consists of two pages. On the right you find the mandala design, the name of the Bach Flower and a channelled message from the respective flower taken from my book *Healing Spirituality–A Practical Guide to Understanding and Working with Bach Flowers*. The parts of the flowers depicted in the illustrations correlate with the parts of the flowers used in the creation of the actual Bach Flower essences. The page to the left of the mandala is the *Reflections* page, a blank page to be used as a journal according to your personal choice. The quotes from Edward Bach on this page have been added to share his spirit and incredible wisdom, both enhancing the experience.

The order of the Bach Flower mandalas might appear random but in fact they are organized according to the numbers each flower resonates to. If you are looking for a specific Bach Flower, the index in the back of the book can help you find it more easily.

"Then I was standing on the highest mountain of them all, and around and about me was the whole hoop of the world...I was seeing in a sacred manner the shapes of all things in the spirit and the shapes of all shapes as they must live together like one being. And I saw that the Sacred Hoop of my people was one of many hoops that made one circle, wide as daylight and starlight and in the centre grew one almighty flowering tree to shelter all the children of one mother and one father, and I saw that it was holy."

~FROM THE VISION OF NICHOLAS BLACK ELK–LAKOTA HOLY MAN: 1863-1950

REFLECTIONS

"And as the Creator, in His mercy, has placed certain Divinely-enriched herbs to assist us to our victory, let us seek out these and use them to the best of our ability, to help us climb the mountain of our evolution, until the day when we shall reach the summit of perfection."

~EDWARD BACH

Star of Bethlehem

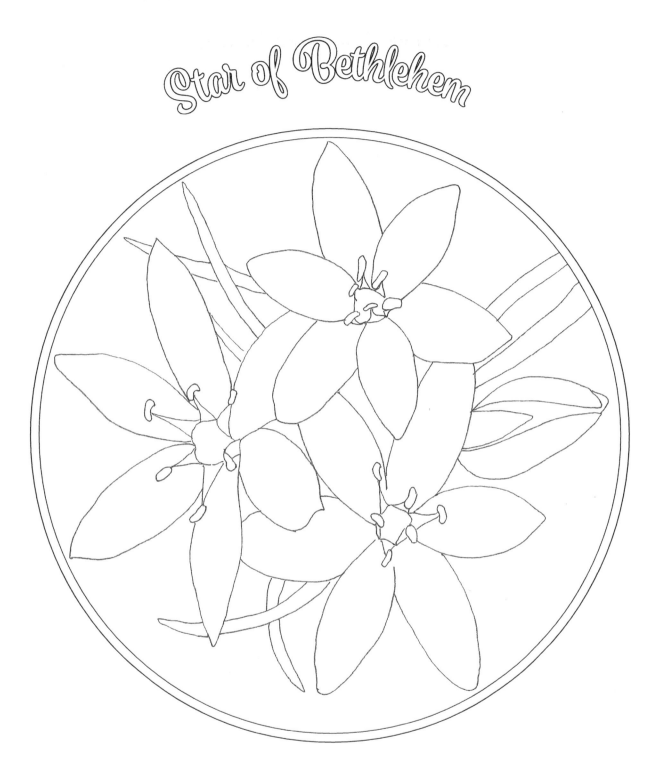

"I, Star of Bethlehem, fill your being with the most gentle and loving essence of hope and healing, releasing from your cellular memory all that does not serve you."

~GUDRUN PENSELIN

REFLECTIONS

"Once we realize our own Divinity the rest is easy."

~EDWARD BACH

Cerato

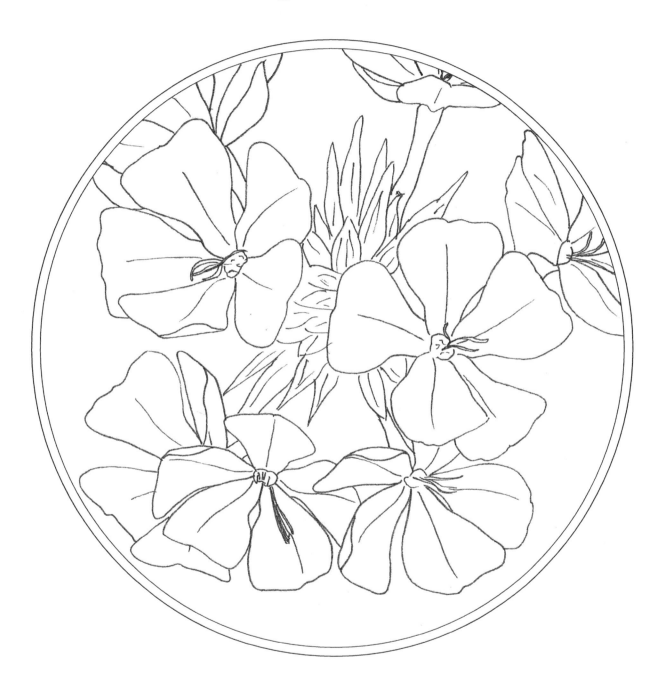

"I, Cerato, guide you so that you may walk with confidence on this Earth, radiating all you know and dwelling in the energies of frequencies of light."

~GUDRUN PENSELIN

REFLECTIONS

"Thus every personality we meet in life, whether mother, husband, child, stranger or friend, becomes a fellow-traveller, and any of them may be greater or smaller than ourselves as regards spiritual development; but all of us are members of a common brotherhood and part of a great community making the same journey and with the same glorious end in view."

~EDWARD BACH

Heather

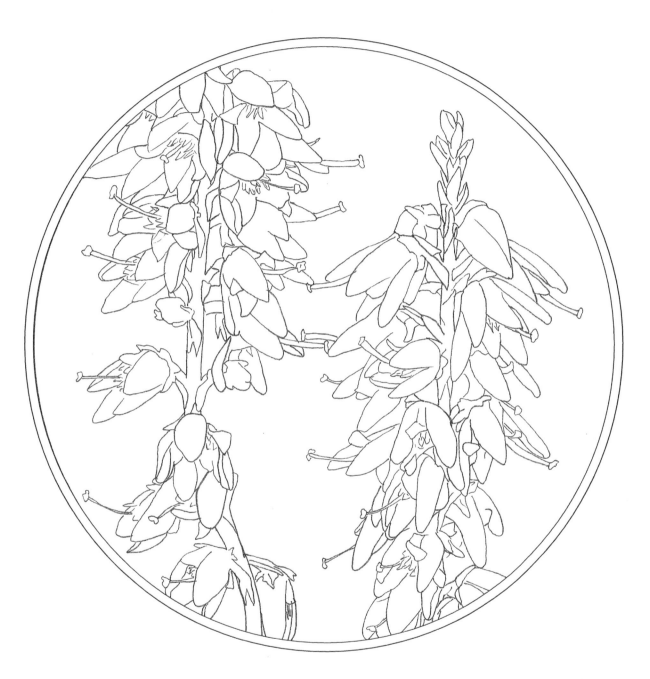

"I, Heather, am strengthening your connection to your true Soul essence, creating a sense of peace and comfort within yourself."

~GUDRUN PENSELIN

REFLECTIONS

"It is in the simple things of life – the simple things because they are nearer the great Truth that real pleasure is to be found."

~EDWARD BACH

White Chestnut

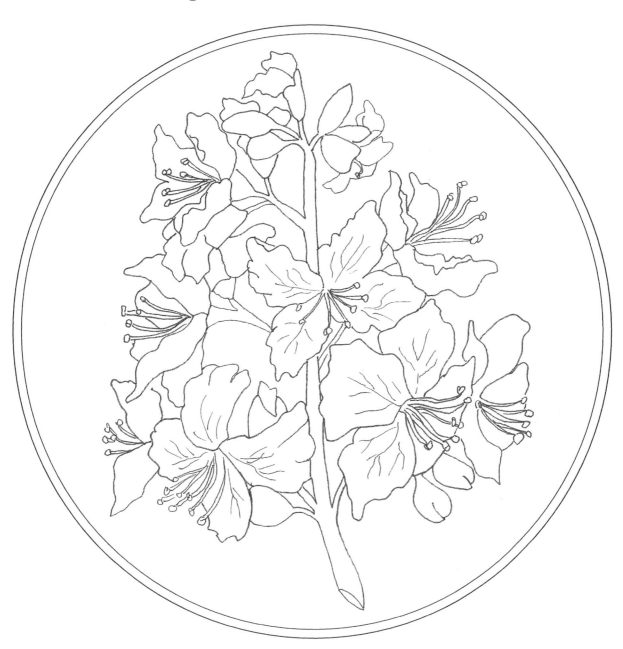

"I, White Chestnut, bring forth a magnificent light to fill your being. Breathe in this light and like a gentle breeze it will cleanse your mind, creating focus and peace of mind."

~GUDRUN PENSELIN

REFLECTIONS

.

"Not one of us upon this earth is being asked to do more than is within his power to perform, and if we strive to obtain the best within us, ever guided by our Higher Self, health and happiness is a possibility for each one."

~EDWARD BACH

Sweet Chestnut

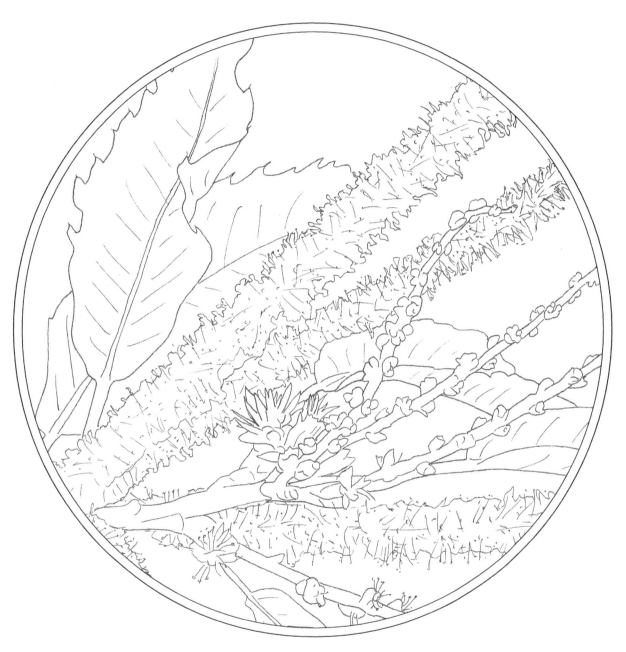

"I, Sweet Chestnut, enlighten your being, sharing my love and light freely with you. Take a deep breath, step back and relax so you can clearly see the light at the end of the tunnel."

~GUDRUN PENSELIN

REFLECTIONS

"Every kindly smile, every kindly thought and action; every deed done for love or sympathy or compassion of others proves that there is something greater within us than what we see. That we carry a Spark of the Divine, that within us resides a Vital and Immortal principle."

~EDWARD BACH

Red Chestnut

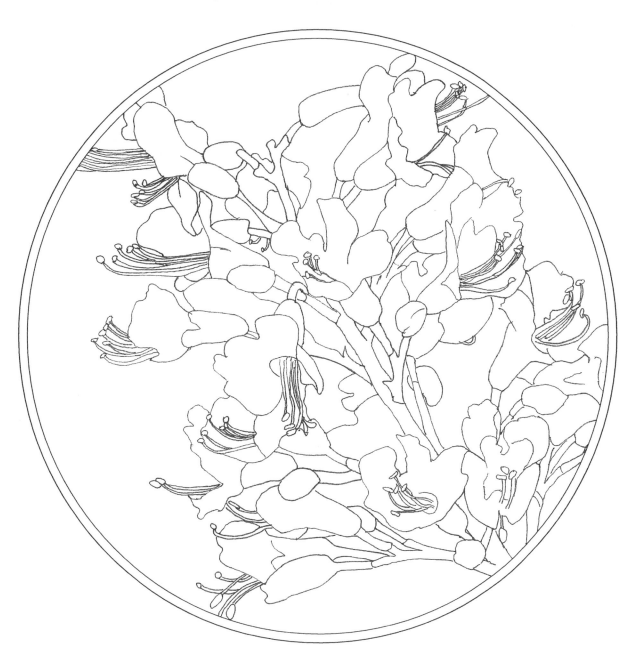

*"I, Red Chestnut, encourage balance and harmony in your life by radiating clarity
and understanding, transforming imbalances into love and light energy."*

~GUDRUN PENSELIN

REFLECTIONS

"As long as we follow the path laid down by the soul, all is well; and we can further rest that in whatever station of life we are placed, princely or lowly, it contains the lessons and experiences necessary at the moment for our evolution, and gives us the best advantage for the development of ourselves."

~EDWARD BACH

Wild Oat

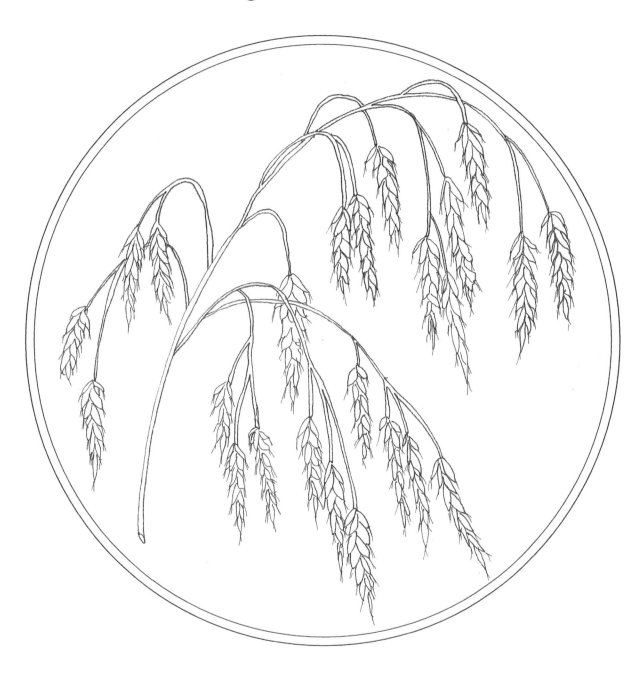

"Feel my energy like the touch of a gentle breeze, stroking you with the essence of light, illuminating your being, bringing clarity and guidance to your Soul."

~GUDRUN PENSELIN

REFLECTIONS

"We should strive to be so gentle, so quiet, so patiently helpful that we move among our fellow men more as a breath of air or a ray of sunshine; ever ready to help them when they ask: but never forcing them to our own views."

~EDWARD BACH

Chicory

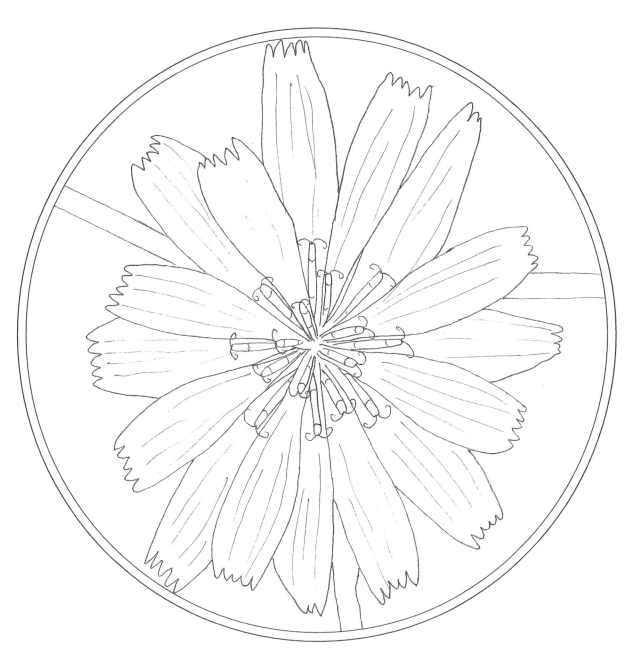

"I, Chicory, fill your energy fields–physical, emotional, esoteric–with my magical, iridescent blue light so that you may experience happiness, peace and harmony arising from within you."

~GUDRUN PENSELIN

REFLECTIONS

"Our soul (the still small voice, God's own voice) speaks to us through our intuition, our instincts, our desires, ideals, our ordinary likes and dislikes; in whichever way it is easiest for us individually to hear."

~EDWARD BACH

Water Violet

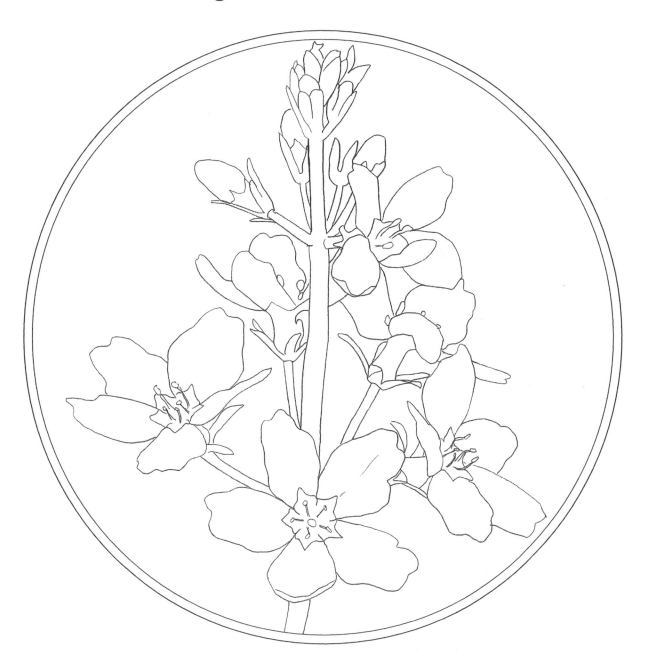

"High frequencies resonate like soft music within you creating peace, harmony and a sense of belonging. This song, I share with you freely. Open your heart and "listen" carefully so that you may receive my healing vibrations."

~GUDRUN PENSELIN

REFLECTIONS

"Thus teach people, as children of the Creator, the Divine individuality within them which is able to overcome all trials and difficulties; help them to steer their ship over the sea of life, keeping a true course and heeding not others; and teach them also ever to look ahead, for, however they may have gone out of their course and whatever storms and tempests they may have experienced, there is always ahead for everyone the harbour of peace and security."

~EDWARD BACH

Centaury

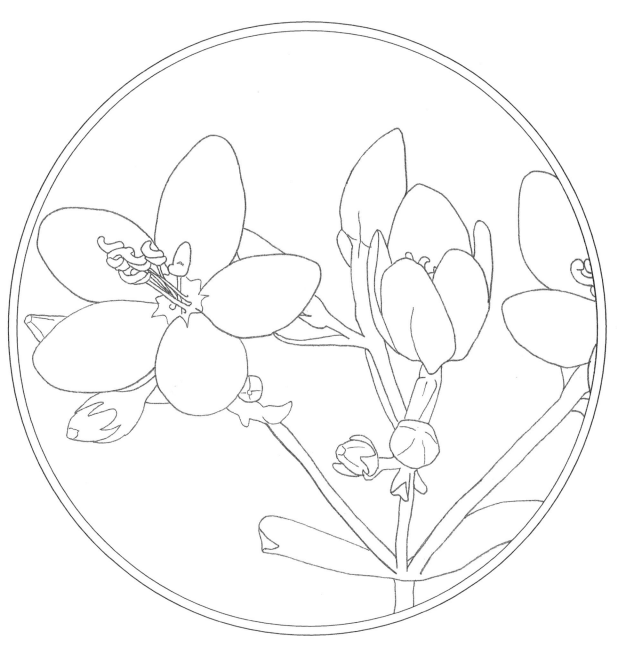

"Soft and gentle I, Centaury, impart trust and courage in you so that giving and receiving are a constant balance of ebb and flow like the waves of the ocean come and go."

~GUDRUN PENSELIN

REFLECTIONS

"Serving through love in perfect freedom in our own way is success, is health."

~EDWARD BACH

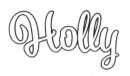

Holly

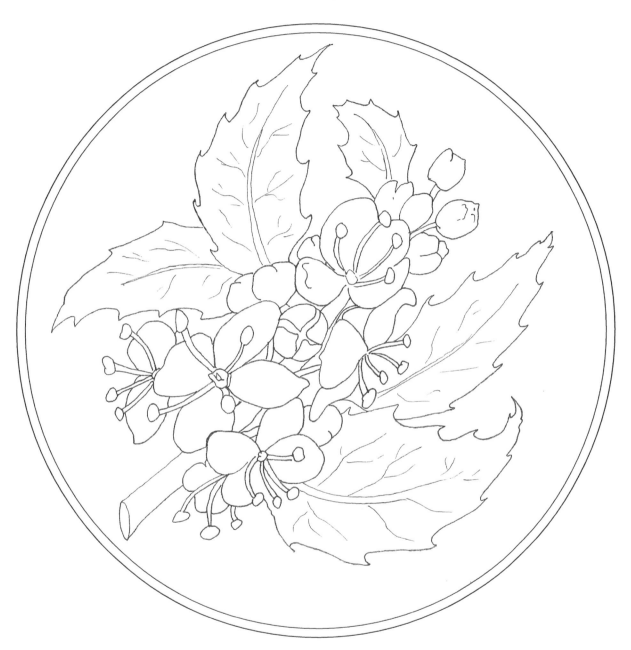

"Breathe deeply; open your heart and trust. Give yourself permission to feel and be filled
with my energies of unconditional love so that every cell of your being radiates golden light,
reflecting acceptance and understanding. Be gentle and loving to self and others."

~GUDRUN PENSELIN

REFLECTIONS

"Nothing in nature can hurt us when we are happy and in harmony, on the contrary all nature is there for our use and our enjoyment."

~EDWARD BACH

Clematis

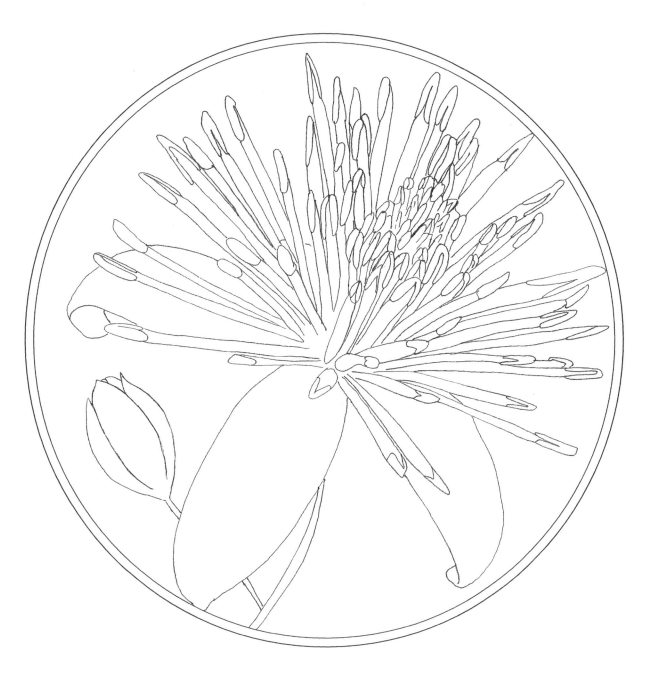

"I, Clematis, bring to you the beautiful vibrations of our Mother Earth guiding you in shifting your focus from dreaming of the "moon and the stars" to who you are and to your direction in life. Be conscious of the moment and you will live your dreams."

~GUDRUN PENSELIN

REFLECTIONS

"They cure not by attacking disease, but by flooding our bodies with the beautiful vibrations of our Higher Nature, in the presence of which disease melts as snow in the sunshine."

~EDWARD BACH

Oak

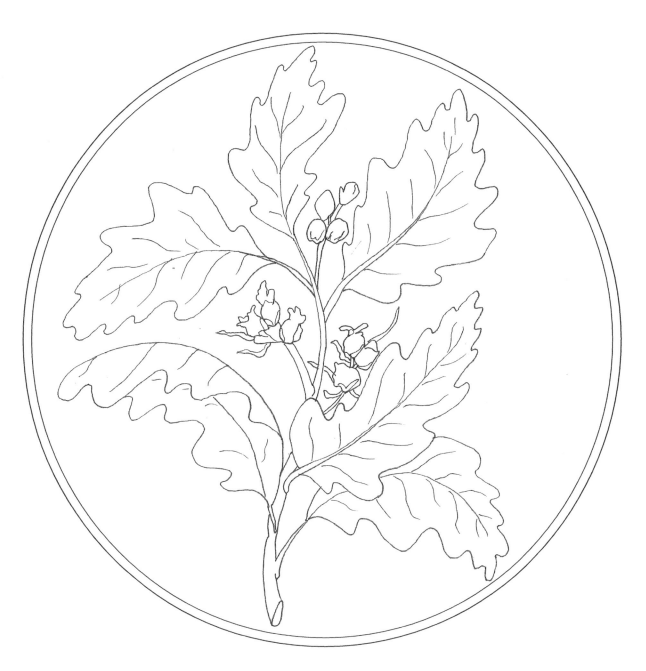

"We, the flowers of the Divine Oak, immerse every cell of your being with our essence, allowing you to feel the power and strength that is inherent to gentleness. Always remember that unconditional love in the form of synchronized balance is the strongest healer of all."

~GUDRUN PENSELIN

REFLECTIONS

"Health depends on being in harmony with our souls."

~EDWARD BACH

Agrimony

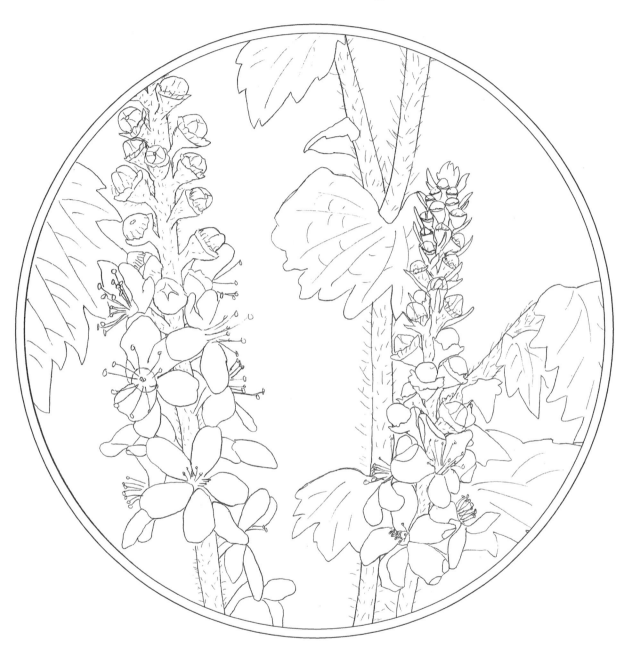

*"I, Agrimony, fill your being with a bright light giving you the
courage to be true to yourself and speak your truth."*

~GUDRUN PENSELIN

REFLECTIONS

"From time immemorial, man has looked at two great sources for Healing. To his Maker, and to the Herbs of the field, which his Maker has placed for the relief of those who suffer."

~EDWARD BACH

Elm

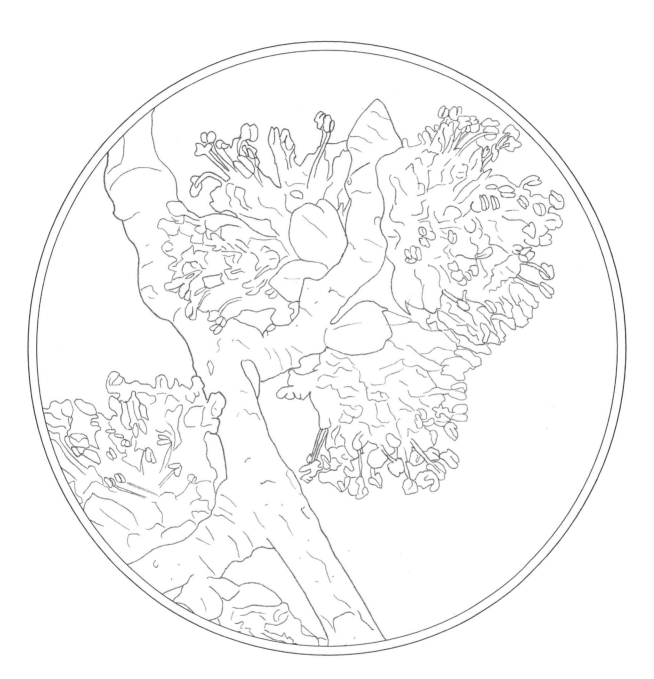

"With synchronized balance, I, Elm, open your channels to the universe to all there is, so that you are able to continue living your Soul essence with courage, optimism, strength and ease. Remember to breathe consciously and deeply."

~GUDRUN PENSELIN

REFLECTIONS

"It is as though in this vast civilization of today, a civilization of great stress and strain, the turmoil has been such that we have become too far parted from the true Source of Healing, Our Divinity."

~EDWARD BACH

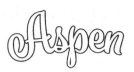

Aspen

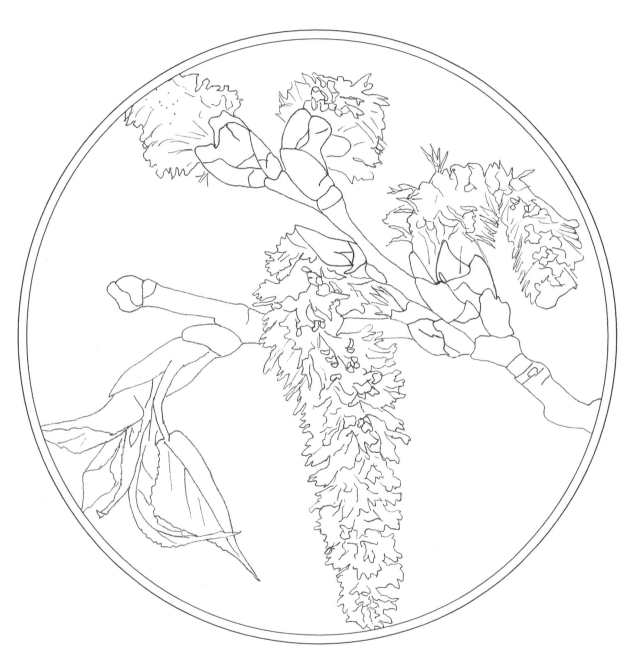

"I, Aspen, am a tree of high frequency. I will shine a bright light, brilliant pearl, bringing transparency and clarity, comfort and ease, enlightening every part of your being."

~GUDRUN PENSELIN

REFLECTIONS

"The amount of peace, of happiness, of joy, of health and of well-being that comes into our lives depends also on the amount of which the Divine Spark can enter and illuminate our existence."

~EDWARD BACH

Wild Rose

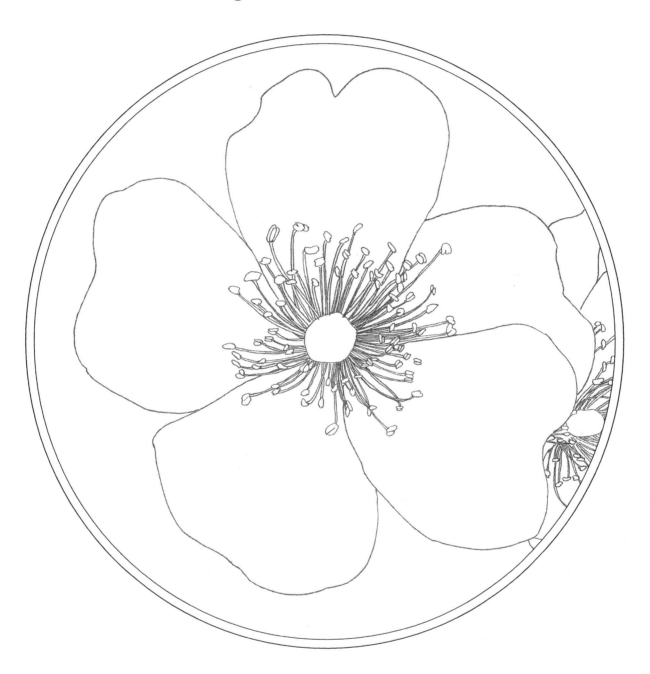

"I am Wild Rose, opening your heart, bringing joy and awareness, guiding you to feel and know that deep within you is what brings joy."

~GUDRUN PENSELIN

REFLECTIONS

*"They are able like beautiful music, or any gloriously uplifting thing which
gives us inspiration, to raise our very natures, and bring us nearer to our Souls:
and by that very act, to bring us peace, and relieve our sufferings."*

~EDWARD BACH

Impatiens

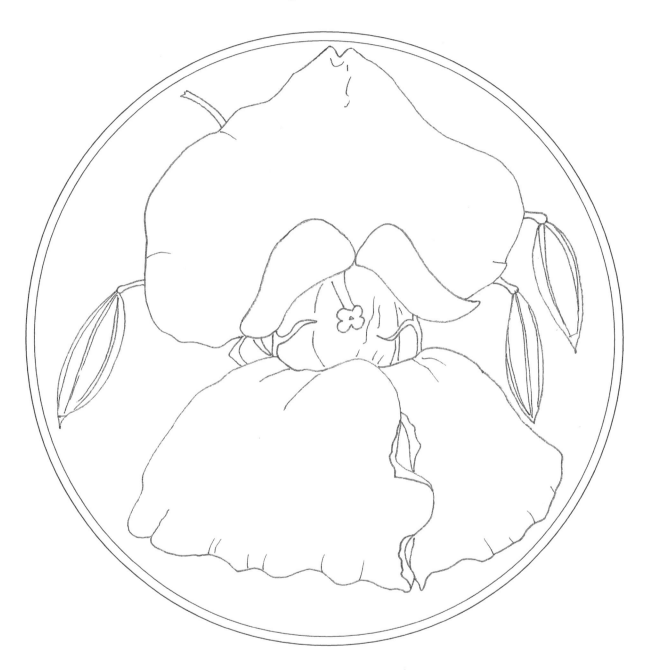

"Open your heart to all aspects of all life within and around you. I, Impatiens, will then flow through you, creating vibrations of understanding and patience leading to peace and harmony."

~GUDRUN PENSELIN

REFLECTIONS

"Simple, natural and gentle acting, the Bach Flower Remedies provide a wonderful tool to help our inherent ability to restore balance and harmony within ourselves."

~EDWARD BACH

Rescue Remedy

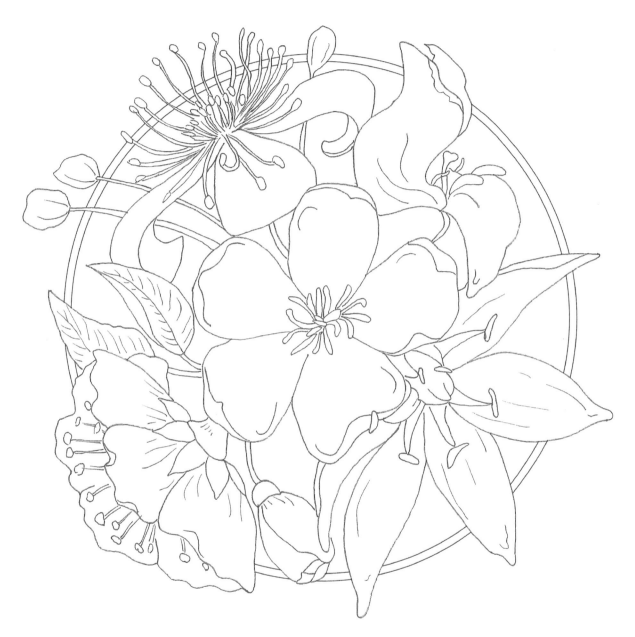

"Breathe deeply and calmly and I will support you in restoring peace and harmony within you by filling your being with loving light."

~GUDRUN PENSELIN

REFLECTIONS

"... those beautiful remedies, which have been Divinely enriched with healing powers, will be administered, to open up those channels to admit more of the light of the Soul, that the patient may be flooded with healing virtue."

~EDWARD BACH

Cherry Plum

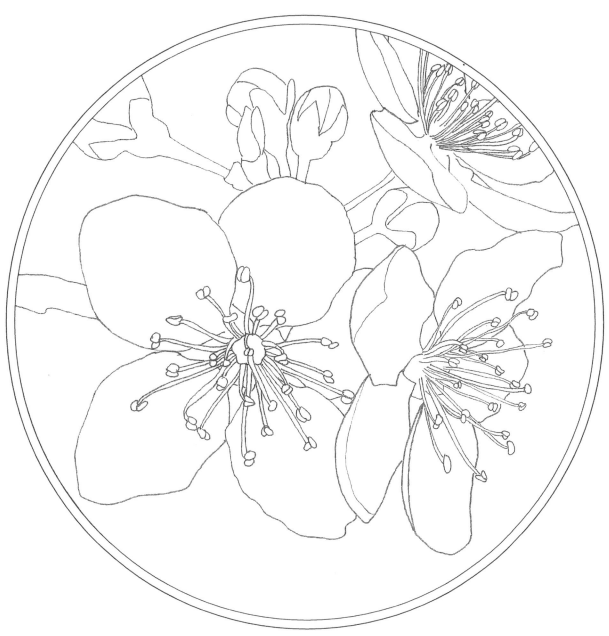

"Breathe my essence in deeply. I, Cherry Plum, assist you in restoring harmony and calmness in your life by transforming fears into trust, synchronized balance and light."

~GUDRUN PENSELIN

REFLECTIONS

*"There are saints at the factory bench and in the stokehold of a ship
as well as among the dignitaries of religious orders."*

~EDWARD BACH

Beech

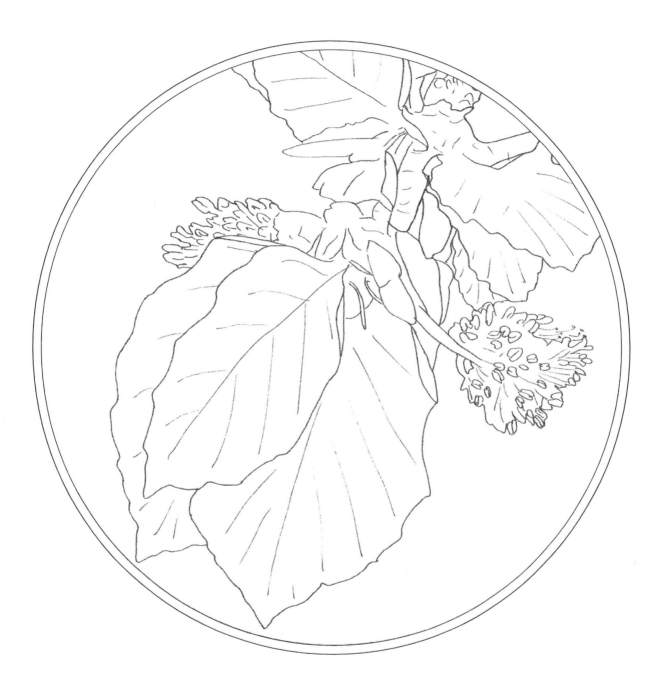

"I, Beech, encourage you to open your heart to my spirit so that you may receive and understand the beauty of acceptance with softness and kindness in all creation within and around you."

~GUDRUN PENSELIN

REFLECTIONS

"Life to him was continuous; an unbroken stream, uninterrupted by what we call death, which merely heralded a change of conditions, and he was convinced that some work could only be done under earthly conditions, whilst spiritual conditions were necessary for certain works."

~NORA WEEKS

Gentian

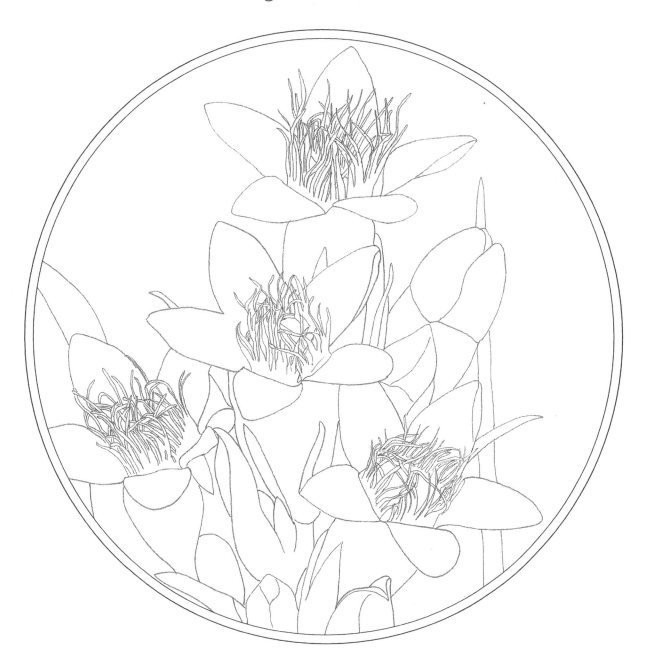

"I, Gentian, am of high vibrational frequency. Like gentle music from the ultimate source, I am filling your being with love and light, encouraging you to move forward with ease."

~GUDRUN PENSELIN

REFLECTIONS

"Let us develop our individuality that we may obtain complete freedom to serve the Divinity within ourselves, and that Divinity alone, and give unto all others their absolute freedom, and serve them as much as lies within our power, according to the dictates of our Souls, ever remembering that as our own liberty increases, so grows our freedom and ability to serve our fellow-men."

~EDWARD BACH

Willow

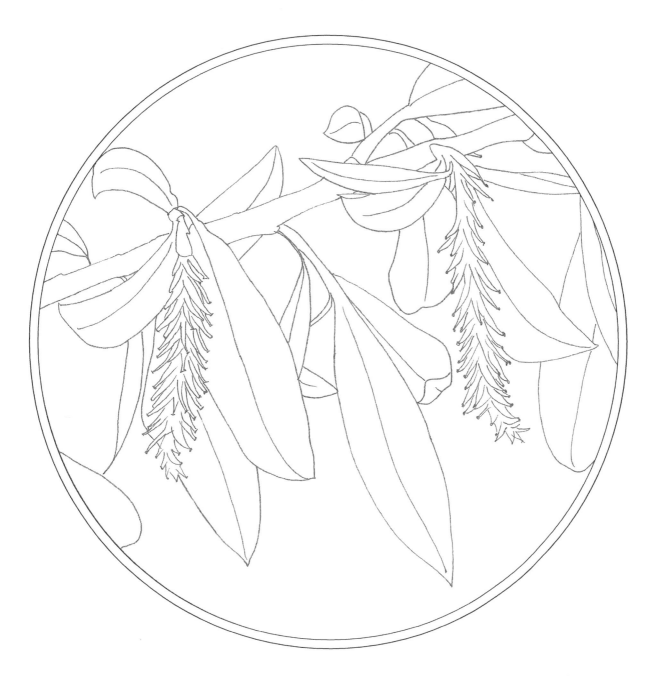

"I, Willow, flood you with synchronized harmony, cleansing all that is not yours and teach you the true meaning of "master of your own destiny". I spark a bright light within you empowering you to live your life energized with passion and intent."

~GUDRUN PENSELIN

REFLECTIONS

"True hate may be conquered by a greater hate, but it can only be cured by love, cruelty may be prevented by a greater cruelty, but only eliminated when the qualities of sympathy and pity have developed, one fear may be lost and forgotten in the presence of a greater fear, but the real cure of fear is perfect courage."

~EDWARD BACH

Rock Rose

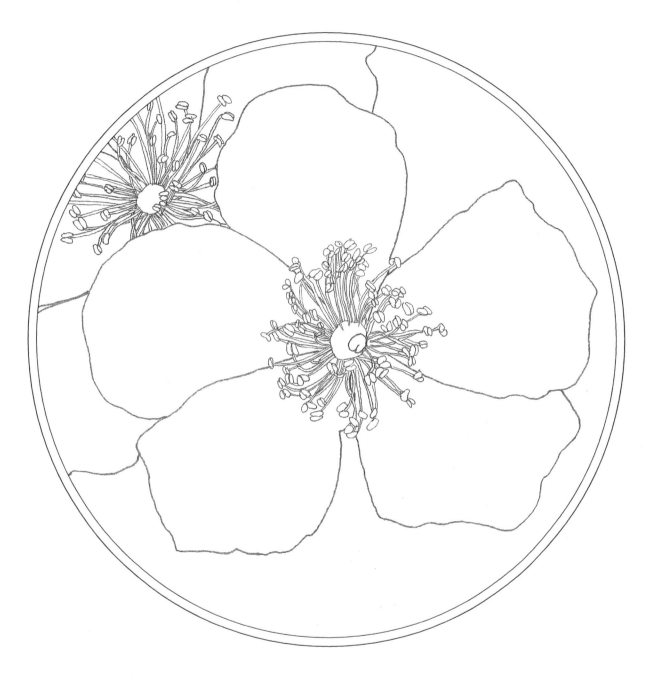

"Trust and I will illuminate your being with golden light, giving you the courage and power to heal."

~GUDRUN PENSELIN

REFLECTIONS

"The whole attitude of parents should be to give the little newcomer all the spiritual, mental and physical guidance to the utmost of their ability, ever remembering that the wee one is an individual soul come down to gain his own experience and knowledge in his own way according to the dictates of his Higher Self, and every possible freedom should be given for unhampered development."

~EDWARD BACH

Pine

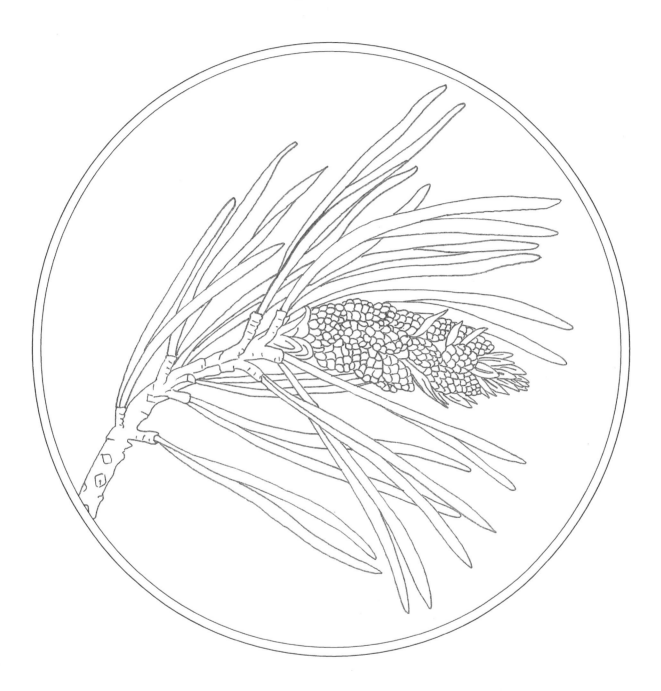

"You were born to manifest the glory of the universe that is within you. Open your heart and you shall receive and understand that perfection is a perception."

~GUDRUN PENSELIN

REFLECTIONS

"These plants are there to extend a helping hand to man in those dark hours of forgetfulness, when he loses sight of divinity, and allows the cloud of fear or pain to obscure his vision."

~EDWARD BACH

Mimulus

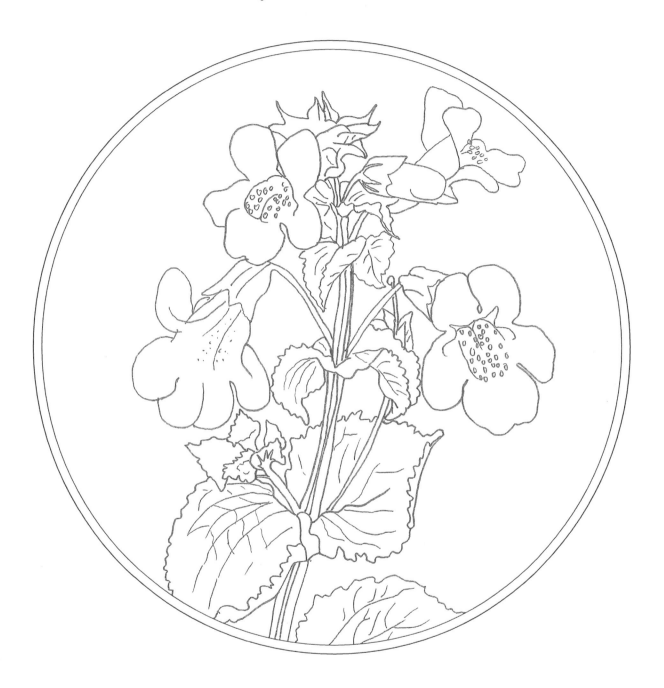

"Trust in me and I will guide you to gently embrace your fears, releasing them to the universe, setting you free and allowing you the freedom to be all who you are meant to be."

~Gudrun Penselin

REFLECTIONS

"Healing must come from within ourselves by acknowledging our faults,
and harmonizing our being with the Divine Plan."

~EDWARD BACH

Crab Apple

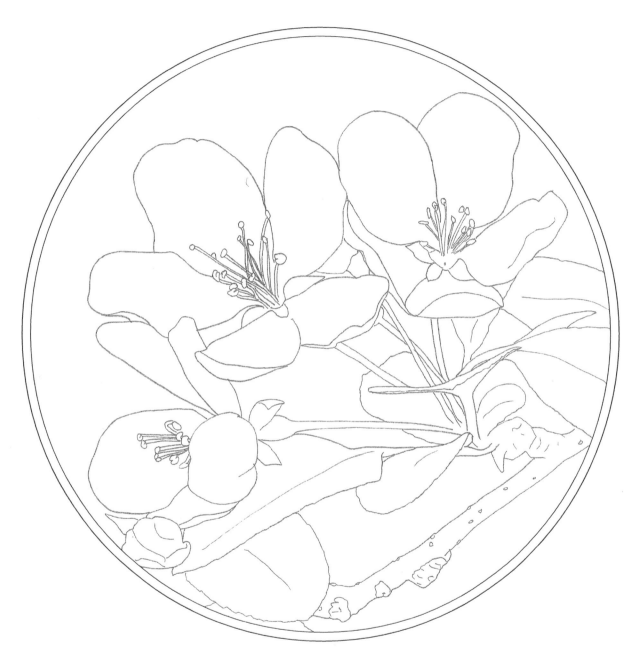

"I, Crab Apple, cleanse all levels of your being by radiating the essence of light and synchronized balance inside of you, allowing you to shift your focus, embrace who you are and heal."

~GUDRUN PENSELIN

REFLECTIONS

"Yet one Truth has mostly been forgotten. That those Herbs of the field placed for Healing, by comforting, by soothing, by relieving our cares, anxieties, bring us nearer to the Divinity within. And it is that increase of the Divinity within which heals us."

~EDWARD BACH

Larch

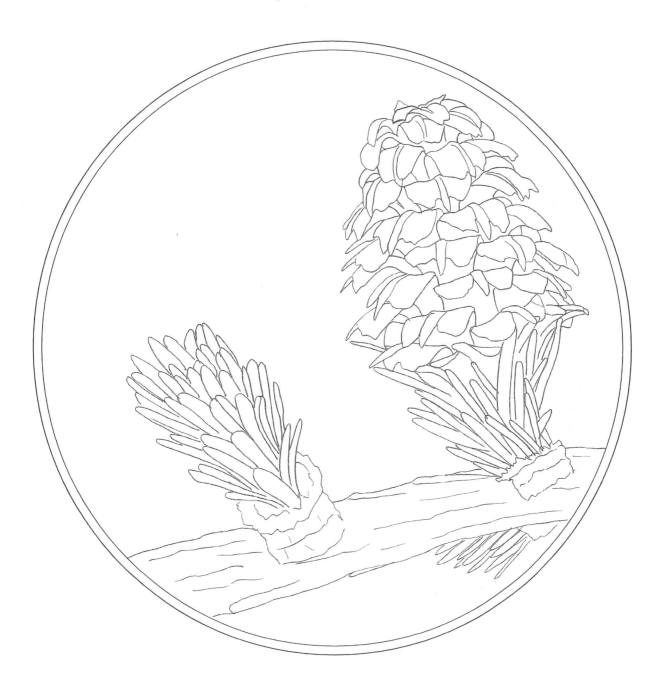

"I, Larch, am here to support you. Trust your inner beauty and abilities and you will discover new shores. Reach for the stars and the moon and watch yourself soar, unfolding to all you can and are meant to be."

~GUDRUN PENSELIN

REFLECTIONS

"Love and Unity are the great foundations of our Creation, ...we ourselves are children of the Divine Love, and ... the eternal conquest of all wrong and suffering will be accomplished by means of gentleness and love."

~EDWARD BACH

Olive

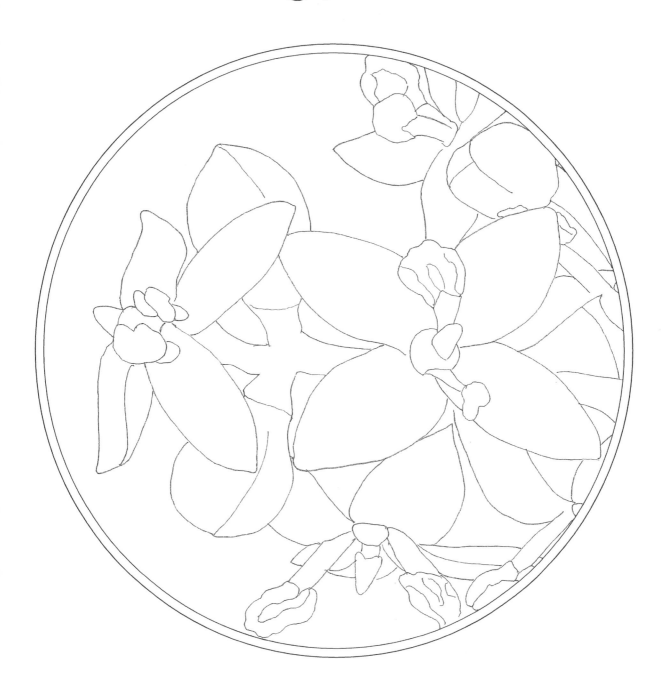

"I am Olive, the fountain of youth, restoring vitality on all levels of your being, while creating peace and harmony."

~Gudrun Penselin

REFLECTIONS

"Every single person has a life to live, a work to do, a glorious personality, a wonderful individuality."
~EDWARD BACH

Walnut

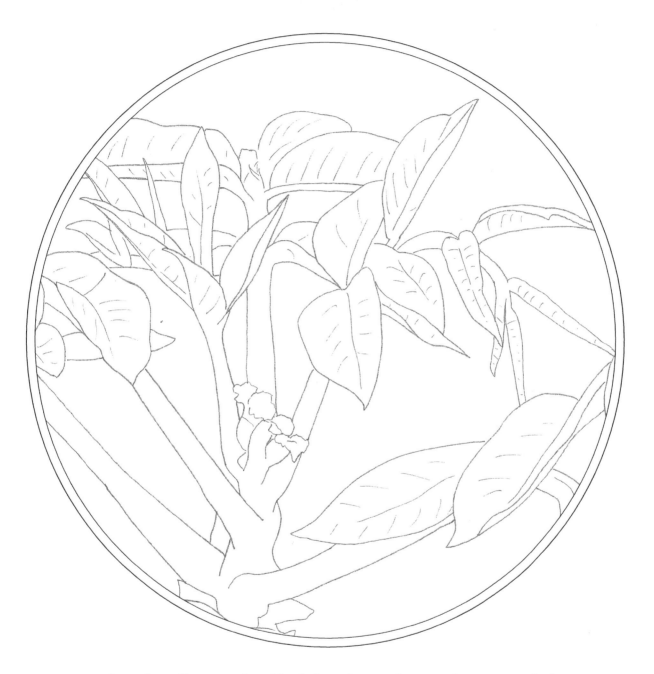

"I, Walnut, illuminate the golden light within you, bringing clarity to your Soul purpose and giving you the strength and determination to be who you are regardless of outside influences. Unfold to your potential and be true to yourself."

~GUDRUN PENSELIN

REFLECTIONS

"Our souls will guide us if we will only listen in every circumstance, every difficulty. The mind and body so directed will pass through life radiating happiness and perfect health."

~EDWARD BACH

Rock Water

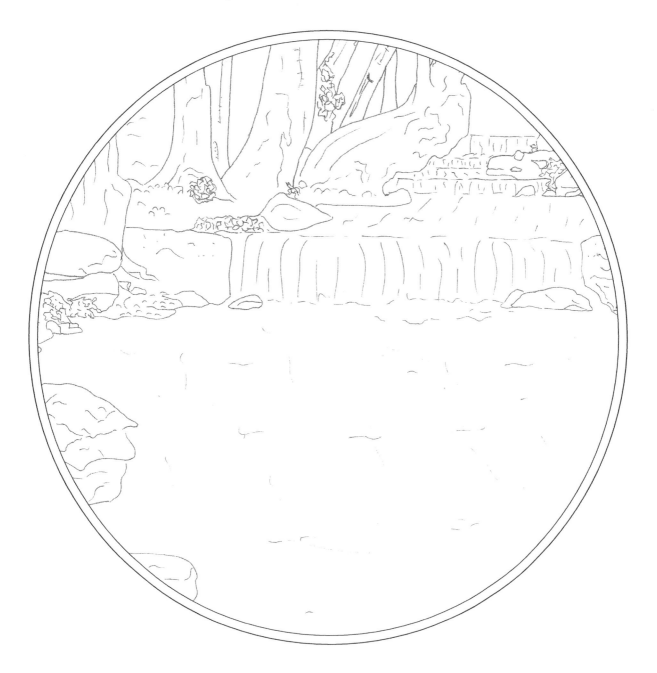

"I, Rock Water, am the spring of life. "Listen" to me with your heart and follow my guidance so your life will flow with ease like a gentle flowing river, seeing the beauty and joy in every moment of life."

~GUDRUN PENSELIN

REFLECTIONS

"Health is our heritage, our right. It is the complete and full union between soul, mind and body; and this is not difficult to attain, but one so easy and natural that many of us have overlooked it."

~EDWARD BACH

Chestnut Bud

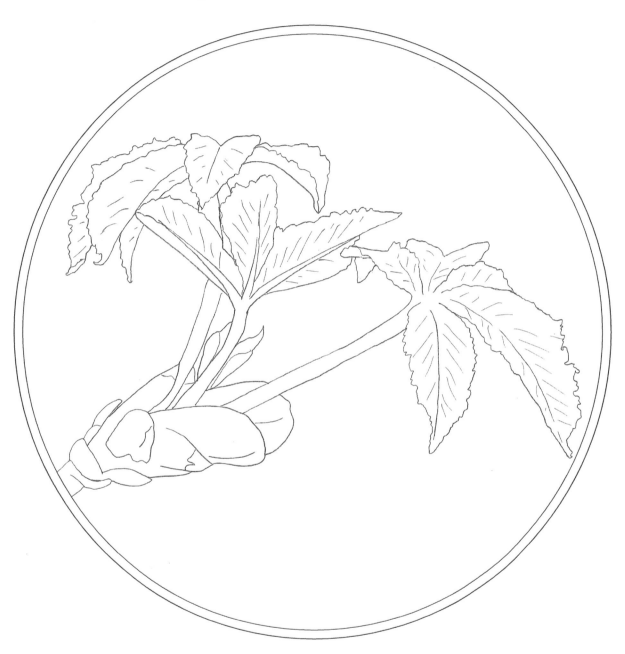

"I, Chestnut Bud, bring consciousness to every moment of your life and guide you to understand the purpose of your experiences that create possibilities for growth and new goals."

~GUDRUN PENSELIN

REFLECTIONS

"To Nature we look confidently for all the needs to keep us alive – air, light, food, drink, and so on, it is not likely that on this great scheme which provides all, the healing of illness and distress should be forgotten."

~EDWARD BACH

Mustard

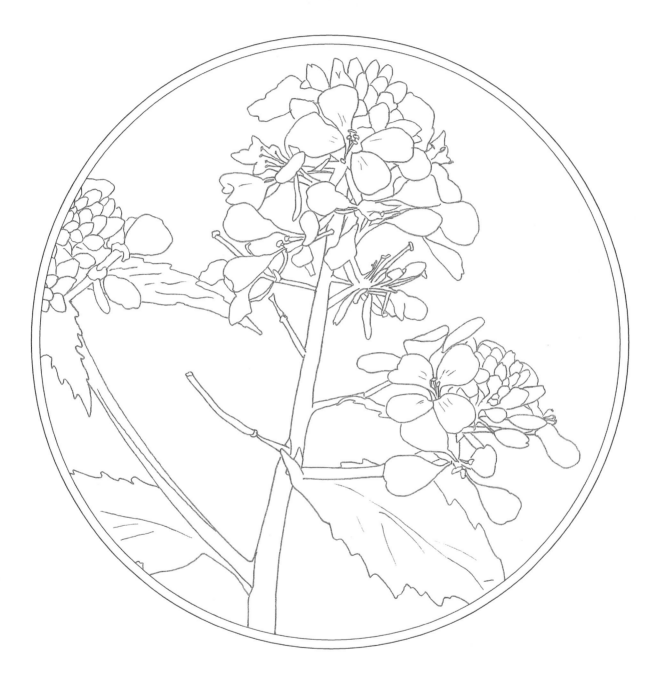

"I, Mustard, am bringing sunshine into your life, absorbing all feelings of despair and hopelessness, lifting your spirit while creating a strong connection to the vibration of universal love."

~GUDRUN PENSELIN

REFLECTIONS

"Never let anyone give up hope of getting well, such wonderful improvements and such marvelous recoveries have happened with the use of these herbs, even in those in which it was considered hopeless that anything could be done; that to despair is no longer necessary."

~EDWARD BACH

Gorse

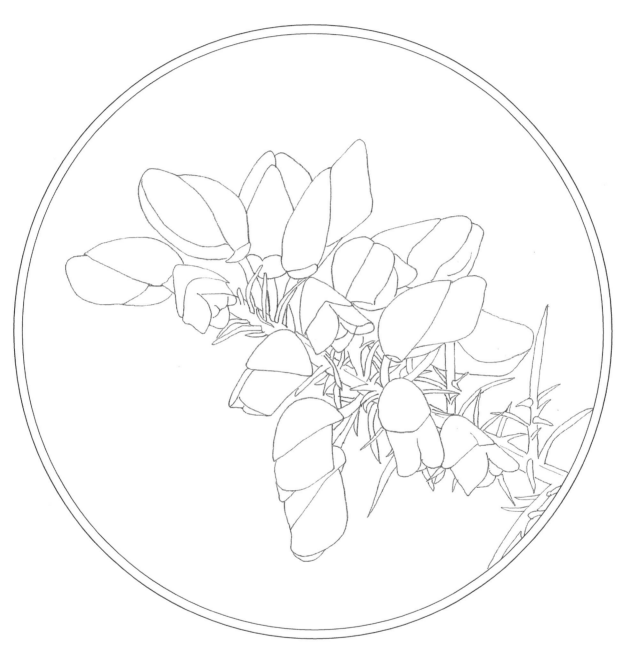

"Open your heart to my vibrations of synchronized balance so that this energy may flow freely through you, transforming darkness into light, filling your being with hope and healing."

~GUDRUN PENSELIN

REFLECTIONS

"The moment that we ourselves have given complete liberty to all around us, when we no longer expect anything from anyone, when our only thought is to give and give and never to take, that moment shall we find that we are free of all the world, our bonds will fall from us, our chains be broken, and for the first time in our lives shall we know the exquisite joy of perfect liberty. Freed from all human restraint, the willing and joyous servant of our Higher Self alone."

~EDWARD BACH

Vervain

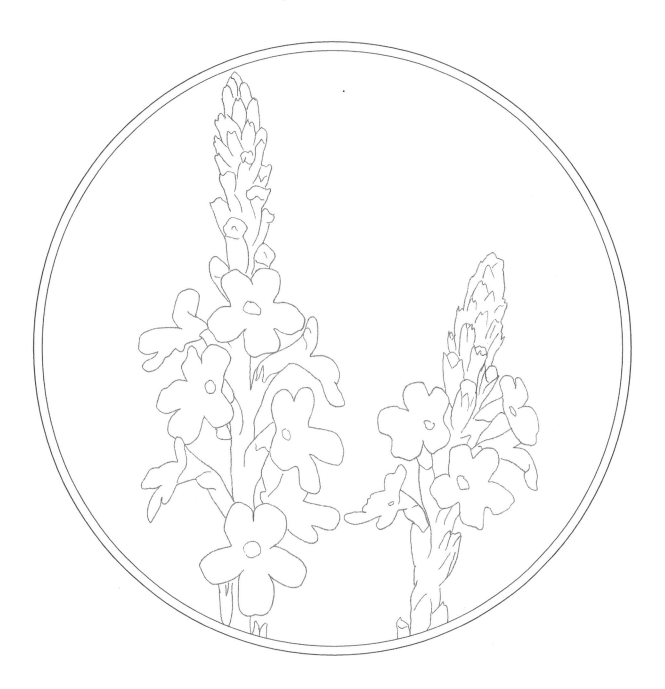

"I, Vervain, fill your being with softness and kindness. I share with you the understanding that knowing your truth is a gift but that not everyone shares the same truth."

~GUDRUN PENSELIN

REFLECTIONS

"And so in true healing, and so in spiritual advancement, we must always seek good to drive out evil, love to conquer hate, and light to dispel darkness. Thus must we avoid all poisons, all harmful things, and use only the beneficent and beautiful."

~EDWARD BACH

Honeysuckle

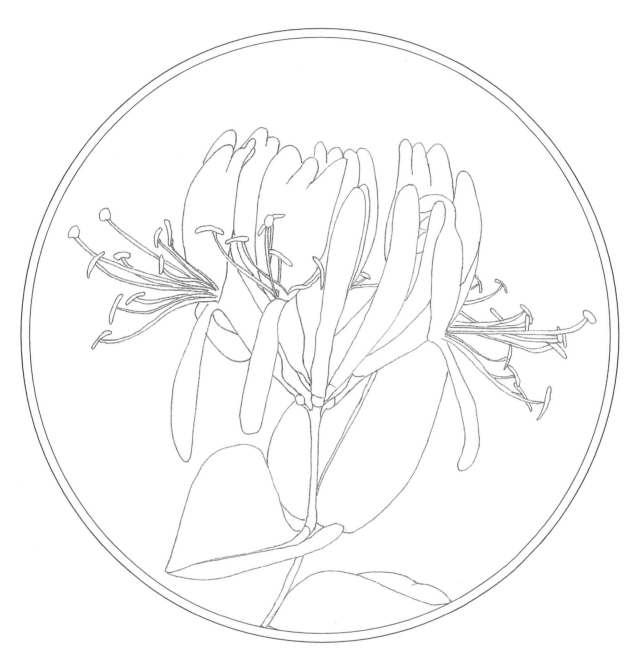

"I, Honeysuckle support your true Soul essence by releasing the past. Sunshine will fill your heart, guiding you to embrace the present."

~GUDRUN PENSELIN

REFLECTIONS

"It must never be forgotten that this (the physical body – author's note) is but the earthly habitation of the Soul, in which we dwell only for a short time in order that we may be able to contact the world for the purpose of gaining experience and knowledge."

~EDWARD BACH

Hornbeam

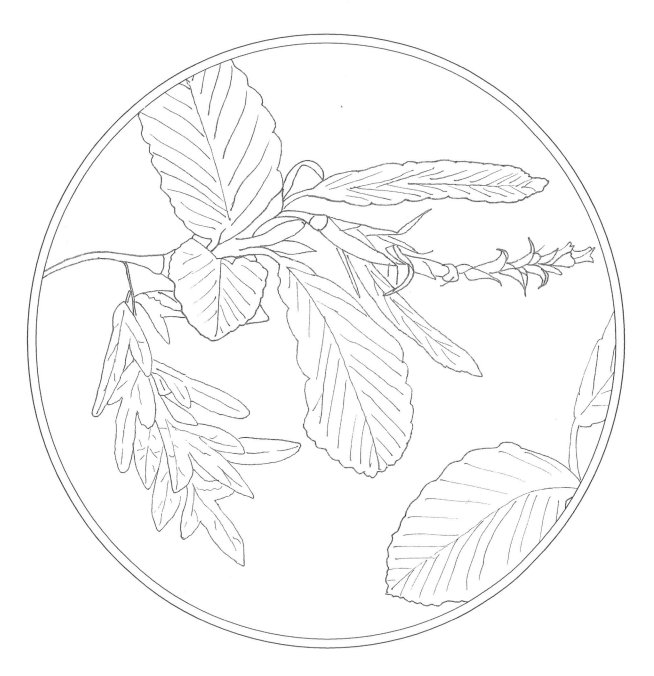

"I, Hornbeam, bring joy and certainty to your life so that all that you have chosen to accomplish will flow with ease in a positive light."

~GUDRUN PENSELIN

REFLECTIONS

"Parenthood is an office in life which passes from one to another, and is in essence a temporary giving of guidance and protection for a brief period, after which time it should then cease its efforts and leave the object of its attention free to advance alone."

~EDWARD BACH

Vine

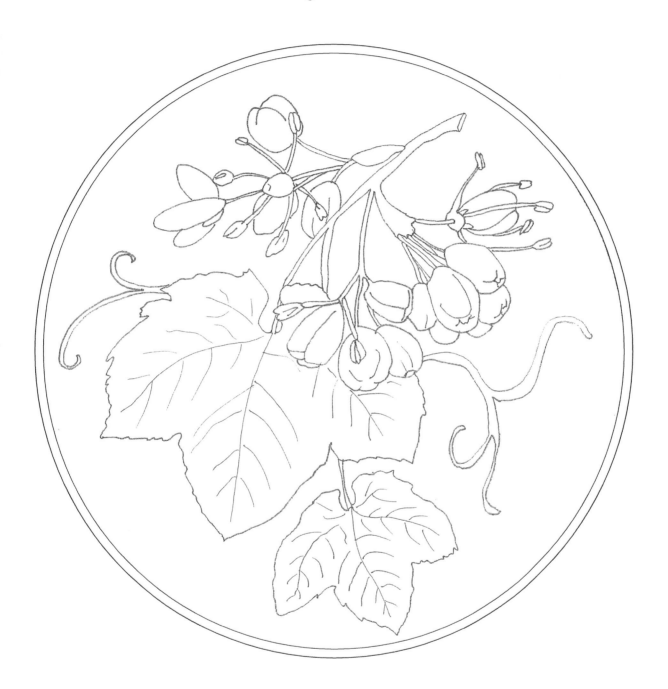

"Be strong but gentle and open your heart towards others, assisting them in seeing and understanding new levels of awareness and consciousness."

~Gudrun Penselin

REFLECTIONS

"Simplicity is the key to all creation."

~EDWARD BACH

Scleranthus

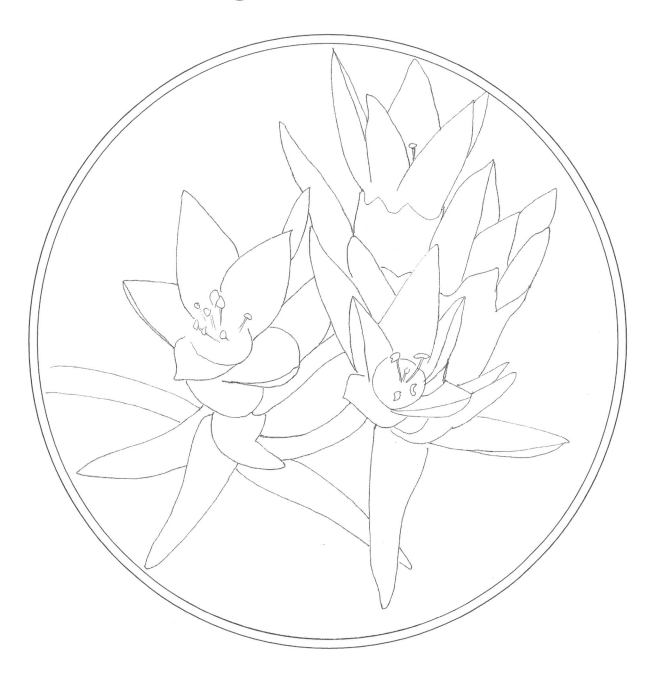

"I, Scleranthus, will simplify your life by giving you clear direction, making it easy for you to walk with great confidence on this Earth."

~GUDRUN PENSELIN

Appendix

If you desire to learn more about Edward Bach and the Bach Flowers you will find a wealth of beneficial, practical information and tools in any of the following publications. All publications are available from Rainbow Healing Publishing, Alberta, Canada.

Healing Spirituality–A Practical Guide to Understanding and Working with Bach Flowers by Gudrun Penselin

"Gudrun Penselin has created a comprehensive and insightful work on the inherent healing qualities of Bach Flowers in HEALING SPIRITUALITY. Flush with historical insight, practical guidance and a thorough understanding of the vibrational healing powers of Bach Flowers, this book is a must-read for both beginners in the field as well as experts, who will benefit from an enriched understanding of remedial flower therapies."

~**STEVEN K. H. AUNG**, *CM AOE MD PhD FAAFP*
Clinical Professor, Faculty of Medicine and Dentistry
Adjunct Professor, Faculties of Extension, Pharmacy & Pharmaceutical
Sciences and Rehabilitation Medicine and School of Public Health
University of Alberta, Edmonton, Alberta, Canada

Healing Spirituality serves as a **practical guide** and **working tool** for the implementation of Bach Flowers into a person's daily life. Edward Bach's original work has been carefully preserved, but the increase in the vibrational frequencies of the Earth affects the information and healing potential brought forth by the Bach Flowers. Therefore, the information has been adjusted to the changes occurring on the planet at this time.

This valuable handbook includes:

- The system of Bach Flowers explained in detail
- Bach Flowers and vibrational healing
- Edward Bach's life, beliefs and philosophy of life and healing
- Detailed description of all Bach Flowers
- Working guide and practical information on how to integrate Bach Flowers into your daily lifestyle
- Instructions for creating your own Bach Flower essences
- and more

Bach Flowers Unfolding by Gudrun Penselin

"The marvellous deck of cards you created, BACH FLOWERS UNFOLDING are a gift one can keep opening and a tool of transformation, in the sense that they bring us into complete harmony with our own intrinsic essence by removing self imposed limitations and helping us access our potential as human beings. To live in a state of balance is a blessing, because it is from this place that we can be truly of benefit to others in our lives. In so doing, the BACH FLOWERS UNFOLDING cards are real friends, assisting us on the path of healing, wherever we are. Your work is very inspiring indeed, Gudrun! Thank you so much for the wisdom they carry, and for their beauty."

~MARGRITH SCHRANER

Bach Flowers Unfolding is a unique and practical tool for working with the Bach Flowers. The essence of the Bach Flowers has been carefully preserved. I was guided to write *Bach Flowers Unfolding,* adjusting the information brought forth by the Bach Flower essences to the higher vibrational frequencies of the Earth, its elements and humankind. The cards can be used on their own or in addition to the actual Bach Flower essences.

Bach Flowers Unfolding includes a deck of cards, one for each Bach Flower, and a booklet explaining the use of the cards. The booklet also contains information on the use of the actual remedies.

This deck of cards gives detailed descriptions about the respective flower essence in regard to the present state of mind and emotional circumstances a person is experiencing as well as the potentially transformed state. Exquisite full colour illustrations enhance the text.

Bach Flowers Unfolding is a practical tool for all ages including the very young for selecting and working with Bach Flower essences.

Herbal Pharmacy for Everyone—A Step-by-Step Guide to Creating Your Own Herbal Preparations

Instructional DVD of over 3 hours with subtitles in English, Spanish, French and German by Gudrun Penselin and Adrian de Landa

"Gudrun and Adrian are each well-schooled in the science of plant medicine but they bring much more to their practice. In refreshing contrast to some current attitudes they bring respect, gratitude and wisdom to the process of harvesting and working with plants. They instruct us to take only what we need and can use at the time, to bring our own calm and loving spirit when we approach and handle plants. And they remind us that all life on this planet is dependent on the plants."

~CATHERINE MCLAUGHLIN

The DVD shares tools of herbal medicine, the most ancient healing art, and provides all the information required to create your own herbal preparations with equipment found in any home kitchen wherever you live.

I have created this DVD out of my concern for the planet and the desire and necessity to provide people with tools that will allow them to take responsibility for their own well-being and at the same time encourage them to re-connect with nature.

The DVD includes the following topics:

- Harvesting, drying and storing herbs
- Demonstration of creation of herbal preparations: juices, water extractions, tinctures, vinegars, **flower essences,** infused oils, ointments, powders and capsules, poultices, fomentations and compresses, steam inhalations, foot and hand baths and more.
- A supplement on how to make your own seed and nut milks as well as sprouting instructions.
- Appendix with formulas and precise instructions.

Bibliography

Cornell, Judith. *The Mandala Healing Kit.* Boulder, Colorado, USA: Sounds True, 2005.

Fincher, Susanne F. *The Mini Mandala Coloring Book.* Boston, Massachusetts, USA: Shambhala Publications, Inc., 2014.

Penselin, Gudrun. *Healing Spirituality–A Practical Guide to Understanding and Working with Bach Flowers.* Wembley, Alberta, Canada: Rainbow Healing Publishing, 2016.

Alphabetical Index of Bach Flowers

Gudrun Penselin

"I see her (Gudrun) as a healer and friend to those around her and the Earth itself, and am constantly inspired to strengthen my own commitment to living a life based in Love... and the singular dedication to the much needed healing of the Earth and its people."

~LANA ROBINSON, B.A., PRESIDING CLERK OF CANADIAN FRIENDS SERVICE COMMITTEE (CFSC)

Gudrun Penselin, M.Ed., is an author, speaker and expert in herbal medicine. She often conducts workshops on herbal pharmacy, connecting to plant spirit, reflexology, light and colour therapy, lifestyle improvement and, of course, the Bach Flowers.

Gudrun has written articles on several topics including medicine making with dried herbs, using Wild Rose and Rosehips for food and medicine, encouraging healing with Bach Flowers, and connecting to the Earth. She is the executive producer and co-creator of the instructional DVD *Herbal Pharmacy for Everyone, A Step-by-Step Guide to Creating Your Own Herbal Preparations* and created the *Bach Flowers Unfolding* card deck.

Gudrun is a natural educator who brings joy whenever she shares her knowledge and experience about plants and their healing spirit. She is a frequent presenter at conferences in Canada and the US and has been a featured guest on numerous radio shows.

Gudrun was born and raised in Germany. Since her emigration to Canada in 1981, she has focused her professional education on complementary medicine. For over 30 years she has been running a successful practice in Grande Prairie, Alberta. She has helped thousands of people through her teachings and practice by using a holistic approach to wellness.

She enjoys the outdoors and being close to nature. Gudrun has explored many parts of Canada with her family while camping, canoeing and hiking in the wilderness. Her deep interest in learning about other cultures and their healing traditions led her to travel to many places across the globe, including India, where she was fortunate to spend some time with Mother Teresa. More recently, her travels have taken her to Central and South America, where she focused her attention on some of the traditional forms of healing.

Gudrun Penselin, M.Ed., M.Phys.Ed.Clinical Herbal Therapist Bach Flower PractitionerCertified Reflexologist–Certified Iridologist/Sclerologist — Light-/Colour Therapist

For more information about Gudrun's work, visit
www.rainbowhealing.ca, www.herbalinstructions.com and www.healingspirituality.com

Yana-Lee Kratschat

Yana-Lee was born and raised in northern Alberta, Canada where she resides today with her husband, their high spirited daughter Vera, their horses, goats, dogs and cats. Yana-Lee not only loves the animals but indeed she is an "animal whisperer." From a very young age it became evident that Yana-Lee is not only very gifted in communication with animals but that she has also great creative and artistic talents. *Healing with Bach Flower Mandalas* has given her the opportunity to share her talent for the first time on a larger scale.

Made in the USA
Charleston, SC
10 December 2016